Diabetic Vegetables & Soups Cookbook

A Mouth-Watering Collection of Diabetic Vegetable & Soup Recipes

Valerie Blanchard

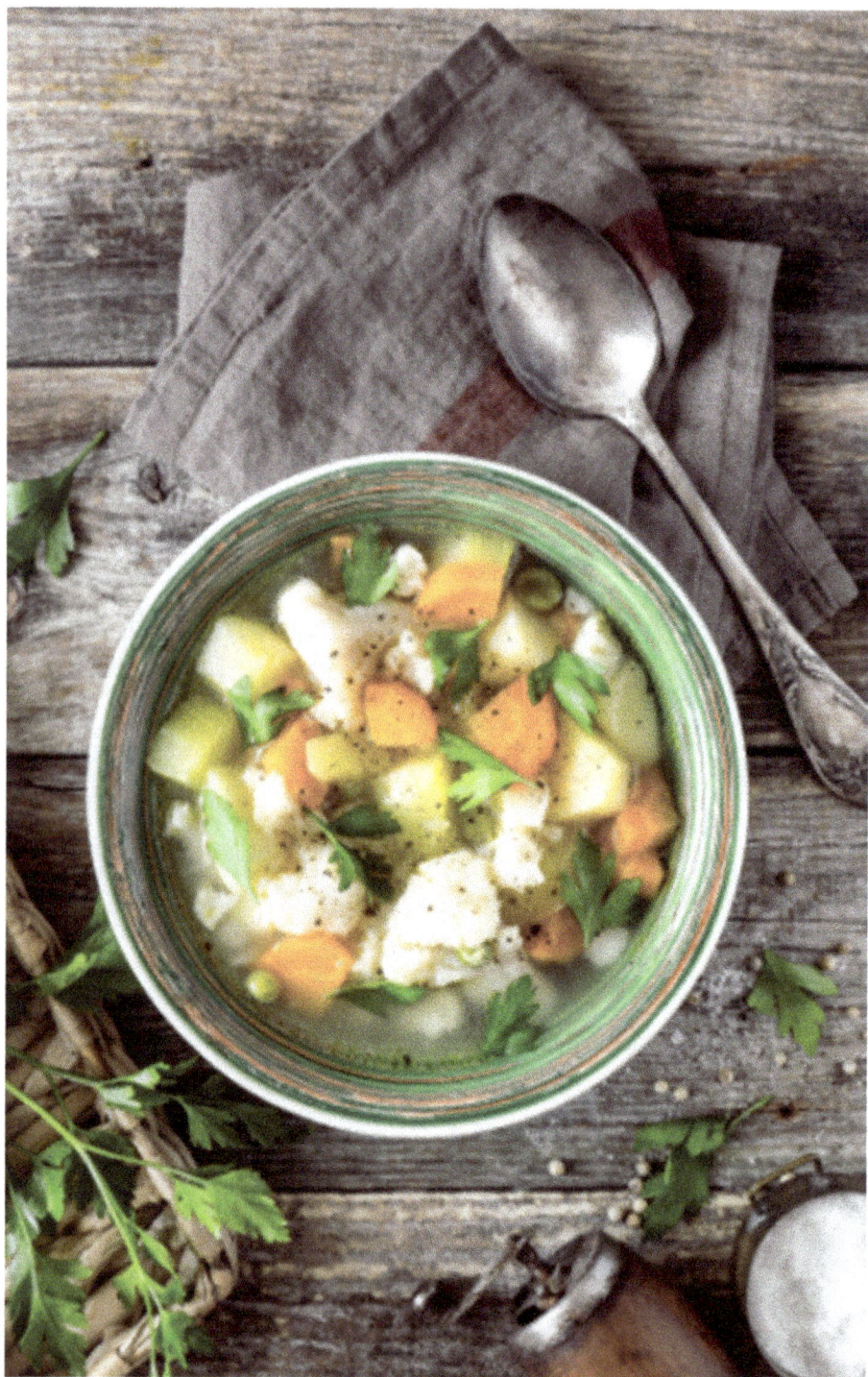

Table of Contents

ROASTED PARSNIPS 7

LOWER CARB HUMMUS 9

SWEET AND SOUR RED CABBAGE 11

PINTO BEANS 14

PARMESAN CAULIFLOWER MASH 16

STEAMED ASPARAGUS 18

SQUASH MEDLEY 20

EGGPLANT CURRY 22

LENTIL AND EGGPLANT STEW 24

TOFU CURRY 25

LENTIL AND CHICKPEA CURRY 27

SPLIT PEA STEW 29

FRIED TOFU HOTPOT 30

CHILI SIN CARNE 31

CHICK PEA AND KALE DISH 32

ZUCCHINI CHIPS 35

CLASSIC BLUEBERRY SPELT MUFFINS 37

GENUINE HEALTHY CRACKERS 39

TORTILLA CHIPS 41

PUMPKIN SPICE CRACKERS 43

SPICY ROASTED NUTS 45

WHEAT CRACKERS 47

POTATO CHIPS 50

ZUCCHINI PEPPER CHIPS 52

APPLE CHIPS 54

KALE CRISPS 56

CARROT CHIPS 58

PITA CHIPS 60

Sweet Potato Chips..62

Spinach and Sesame Crackers 64

Mini Nacho Pizzas...66

Pizza Sticks 68

Raw Broccoli Poppers 70

Blueberry Cauliflower 73

Candied Ginger 75

Chia Crackers 78

Orange- Spiced Pumpkin Hummus..81

Cinnamon Maple Sweet Potato Bites 83

Cheesy Kale Chips 85

Lemon Roasted Bell Pepper 87

Subtle Roasted Mushrooms 89

Fancy Spelt Bread...91

Crispy Crunchy Hummus 93

Dill Celery Soup..95

Creamy Avocado-Broccoli Soup 97

Fresh Garden Vegetable Soup 100

Raw Some Gazpacho Soup...102

Alkaline Carrot Soup with Fresh Mushrooms....................................104

Swiss Cauliflower-Omental-Soup...106

Chilled Parsley-Gazpacho with Lime & Cucumber.............................108

Chilled Avocado Tomato Soup...110

Roasted Parsnips

Preparation Time: 9 minutes

Cooking Time: 25 minutes

Servings: *2*

Ingredients:

- 1lb parsnips
- 1 cup vegetable stock
- 2tbsp herbs
- 2tbsp olive oil

Directions:

1. Put the parsnips in the steamer basket and add the stock into the Instant Pot.
2. Steam the parsnips in your Instant Pot for 15 minutes.
3. Depressurize and pour away the remaining stock.

4. Set to sauté and add the oil, herbs and parsnips.

5. Cook until golden and crisp.

Nutrition: 130 Calories; 14g Carbohydrates; 4g Protein

Lower Carb Hummus

Preparation Time: 9 minutes

Cooking Time: 60 minutes

Servings: *2*

Ingredients:

- 0.5 cup dry chickpeas
- 1 cup vegetable stock
- 1 cup pumpkin puree
- 2tbsp smoked paprika
- salt and pepper to taste

Directions:

1. Soak the chickpeas overnight.
2. Place the chickpeas and stock in the Instant Pot.
3. Cook on Beans 60 minutes.
4. Depressurize naturally.

5. Blend the chickpeas with the remaining Ingredients.

Nutrition: 135 Calories; 18g Carbohydrates; 3g Fat

Sweet and Sour Red Cabbage

Preparation Time: 7 minutes

Cooking Time: 10 minutes

Servings: *8*

Ingredients:

- 2 cups Spiced Pear Applesauce
- 1 small onion, chopped
- ½ cup apple cider vinegar
- ½ teaspoon kosher salt
- 1 head red cabbage

Directions:

1. In the electric pressure cooker, combine the applesauce, onion, vinegar, salt, and cup of water. Stir in the cabbage.
2. Seal lid of the pressure cooker.
3. Cook on high pressure for 10 minutes.

4. When the cooking is complete, hit Cancel and quick release the pressure.

5. Once the pin drops, unlock and remove the lid.

6. Spoon into a bowl or platter and serve.

Nutrition: 91 Calories; 18g Carbohydrates; 4g Fiber

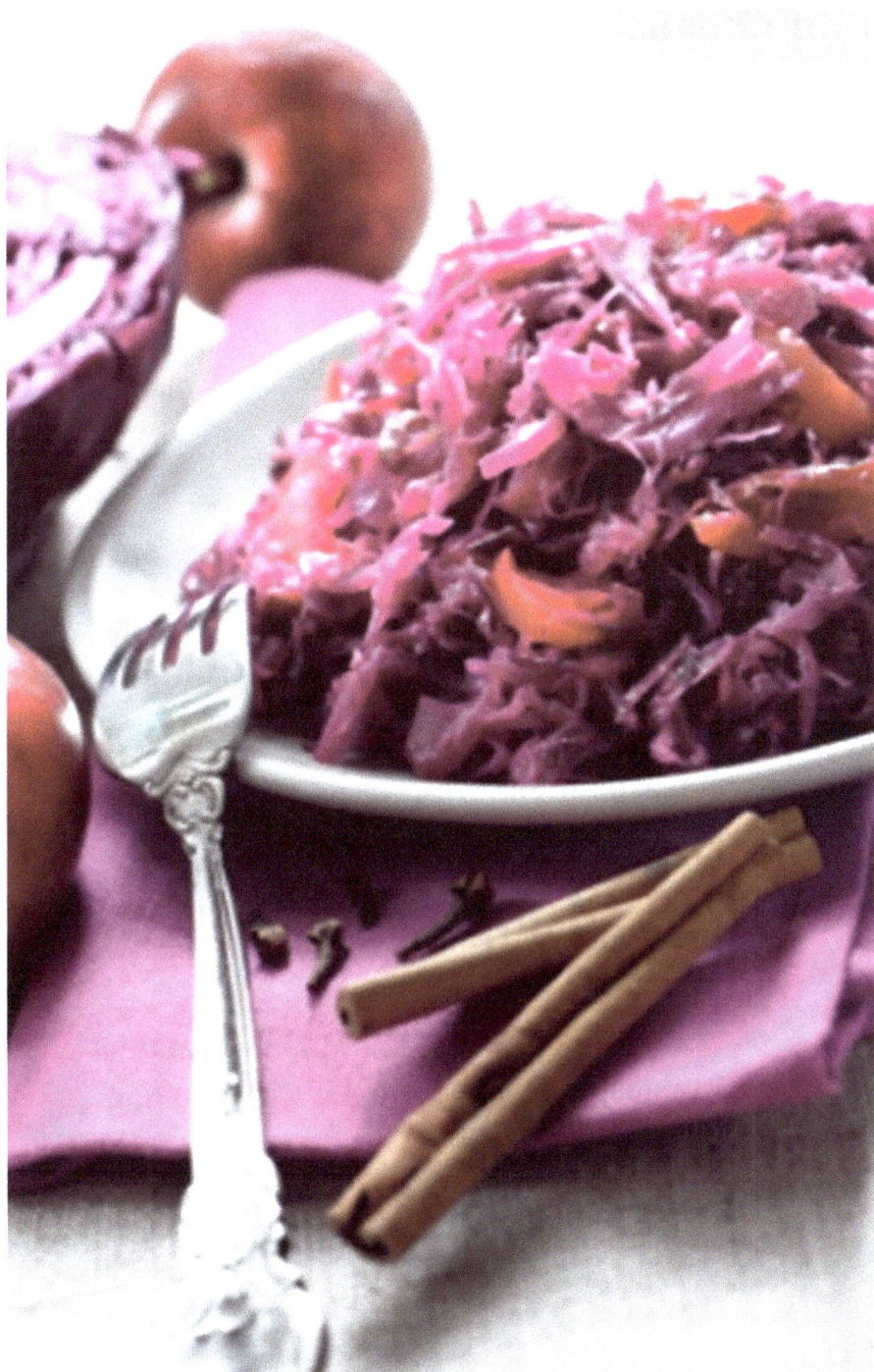

Pinto Beans

Preparation Time: 6 minutes

Cooking Time: 55 minutes

Servings: _10_

Ingredients:

- 2 cups pinto beans, dried
- 1 medium white onion
- 1 ½ teaspoon minced garlic
- ¾ teaspoon salt
- 1/4 teaspoon ground black pepper
- 1 teaspoon red chili powder
- 1/4 teaspoon cumin
- 1 tablespoon olive oil
- 1 teaspoon chopped cilantro
- 5 ½ cup vegetable stock

Directions:

1. Plugin instant pot, insert the inner pot, press sauté/simmer button, add oil and when hot, add onion and garlic and cook for 3 minutes or until onions begin to soften.

2. Add remaining Ingredients , stir well, then press the cancel button, shut the instant pot with its lid and seal the pot.

3. Click 'manual' button, then press the 'timer' to set the Cooking Time to 45 minutes and cook at high pressure.

4. Once done, click 'cancel' button and do natural pressure release for 10 minutes until pressure nob drops down.

5. Open the instant pot, spoon beans into plates and serve.

Nutrition: 107 Calories; 11.7g Carbohydrates; 4g Fiber

Parmesan Cauliflower Mash

Preparation Time: 19 minutes

Cooking Time: 5 minutes

Servings: *4*

Ingredients:

- 1 head cauliflower
- ½ teaspoon kosher salt
- ½ teaspoon garlic pepper
- 2 tablespoons plain Greek yogurt
- ¾ cup freshly grated Parmesan cheese
- 1 tablespoon unsalted butter or ghee (optional)
- Chopped fresh chives

Directions:

1. Pour cup of water into the electric pressure cooker and insert a steamer basket or wire rack.

2. Place the cauliflower in the basket.

3. Cover lid of the pressure cooker to seal.

4. Cook on high pressure for 5 minutes.

5. Once complete, hit Cancel and quick release the pressure.

6. When the pin drops, remove the lid.

7. Remove the cauliflower from the pot and pour out the water. Return the cauliflower to the pot and add the salt, garlic pepper, yogurt, and cheese. Use an immersion blender to purée or mash the cauliflower in the pot.

8. Spoon into a Serving bowl, and garnish with butter (if using) and chives.

Nutrition: 141 Calories; 12g Carbohydrates;4g Fiber

Steamed Asparagus

Preparation Time: 3 minutes

Cooking Time: 2 minutes

Servings: *4*

Ingredients:

- 1 lb. fresh asparagus, rinsed and tough ends trimmed
- 1 cup water

Directions:

1. Place the asparagus into a wire steamer rack, and set it inside your Instant Pot.

2. Add water to the pot. Close and seal the lid, turning the steam release valve to the "Sealing" position.

3. Select the "Steam" function to cook on high pressure for 2 minutes.

4. Once done, do a quick pressure release of the steam.

5. Lift the wire steamer basket out of the pot and place the asparagus onto a **Serving** plate.

6. Season as desired and serve.

Nutrition: 22 Calories; 4g Carbohydrates; 2g Protein

Squash Medley

Preparation Time: 10 minutes

Cooking Time: 20 minutes.

Servings: *2*

Ingredients:

- 2 lbs. mixed squash
- ½ cup mixed veg
- 1 cup vegetable stock
- 2 tbsps. olive oil
- 2 tbsps. mixed herbs

Directions:

1. Put the squash in the steamer basket and add the stock into the instant Pot.

2. Steam the squash in your Instant Pot for 10 minutes.

3. Depressurize and pour away the remaining stock.

4. Set to sauté and add the oil and remaining Ingredients.

5. Cook until a light crust form.

Nutrition: 100 Calories; 10g Carbohydrates; 6g Fat

Eggplant Curry

Preparation Time: 15 minutes

Cooking Time: 20 minutes

Servings: *2*

Ingredients:

- 3 cups chopped eggplant
- 1 thinly sliced onion
- 1 cup coconut milk
- 3 tbsps. curry paste
- 1 tbsp. oil or ghee

Directions:

1. Select Instant Pot to sauté and put the onion, oil, and curry paste.

2. Once the onion is soft, stir in remaining Ingredients and seal.

3. Cook on Stew for 20 minutes. Release the pressure naturally.

Nutrition: 350 Calories; 15g Carbohydrates; 25g Fat

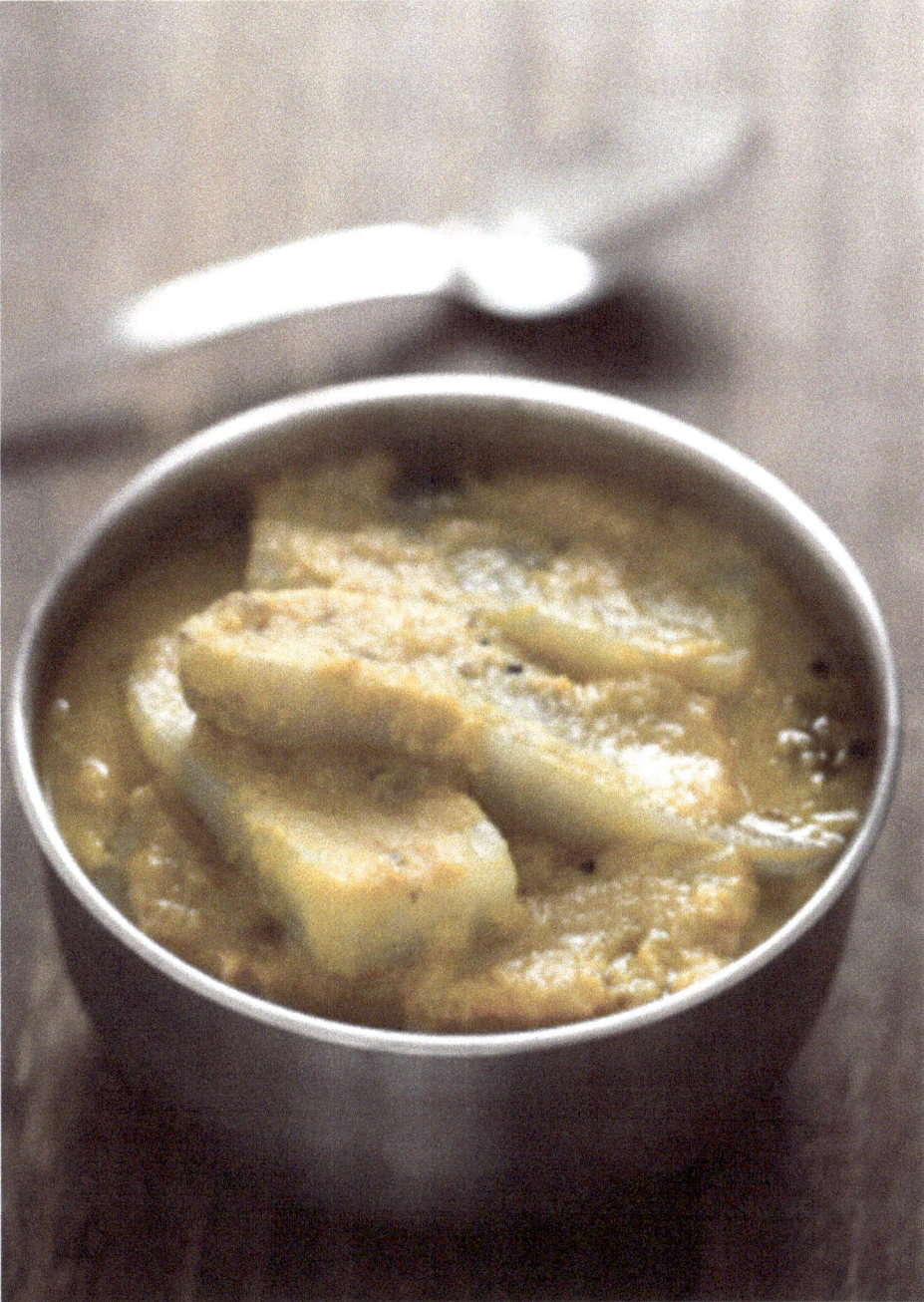

Lentil and Eggplant Stew

Preparation Time: 15 minutes

Cooking Time: 35 minutes

Servings: *2*

Ingredients:

- 1 lb. eggplant
- 1 lb. dry lentils
- 1 cup chopped vegetables
- 1 cup low sodium vegetable broth

Directions:

1. Incorporate all the Ingredients in your Instant Pot, cook on Stew for 35 minutes.
2. Release the pressure naturally and serve.

Nutrition: 310 Calories; 22g Carbohydrates; 10g Fat

Tofu Curry

Preparation Time: 15 minutes

Cooking Time: 20 minutes

Servings: *2*

Ingredients:

- 2 cups cubed extra firm tofu
- 2 cups mixed stir fry vegetables
- ½ cup soy yogurt
- 3 tbsps. curry paste
- 1 tbsp. oil or ghee

Directions:

1. Set the Instant Pot to sauté and add the oil and curry paste.
2. Once soft, place the remaining Ingredients except for the yogurt and seal.
3. Cook on Stew for 20 minutes.

4. Release the pressure naturally and serve with a scoop of soy yogurt.

Nutrition: 300 Calories; 9g Carbohydrates; 14g Fat

Lentil and Chickpea Curry

__Preparation Time:__ 15 minutes

__Cooking Time__: 20 minutes

Servings: *2*

Ingredients:

- 2 cups dry lentils and chickpeas
- 1 thinly sliced onion
- 1 cup chopped tomato
- 3 tbsps. curry paste
- 1 tbsp. oil or ghee

Directions:

1. Press Instant Pot to sauté and mix onion, oil, and curry paste.
2. Once the onion is cooked, stir the remaining Ingredients and seal.
3. Cook on Stew for 20 minutes.

4. Release the pressure naturally and serve.

Nutrition: 360 Calories; 26g Carbohydrates; 19g Fat

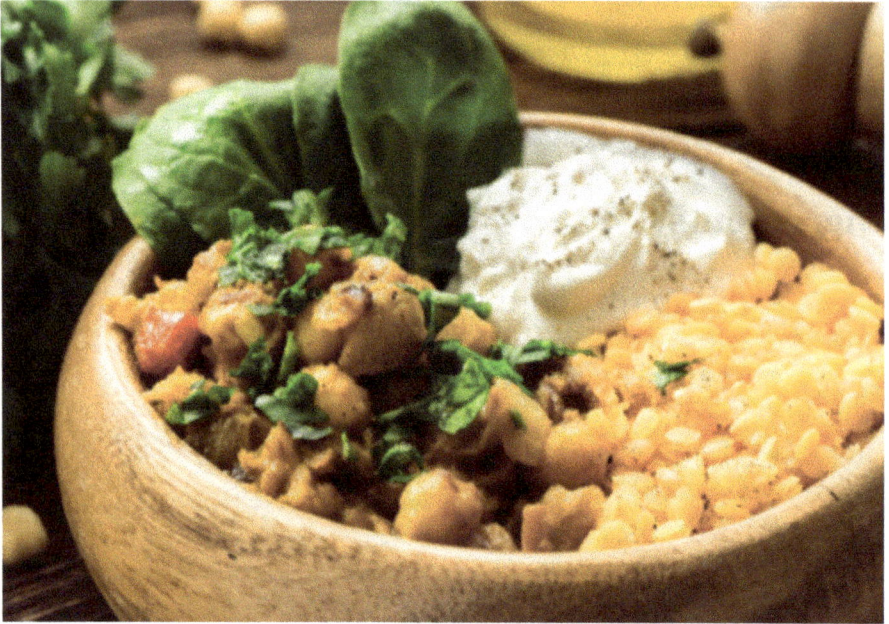

Split Pea Stew

Preparation Time: 5 minutes

Cooking Time: 35 minutes

Servings: *2*

Ingredients:

- 1 cup dry split peas
- 1 lb. chopped vegetables
- 1 cup mushroom soup
- 2 tbsps. old bay seasoning

Directions:

1. Incorporate all the **Ingredients** in Instant Pot, cook for 33 minutes.
2. Release the pressure naturally.

Nutrition: 300 Calories; 7g Carbohydrates; 2g Fat

Fried Tofu Hotpot

Preparation Time: 15 minutes

Cooking Time: 15 minutes

Servings: *2*

Ingredients:

- ½ lb. fried tofu
- 1 lb. chopped Chinese vegetable mix
- 1 cup low sodium vegetable broth
- 2 tbsps. 5 spice seasoning
- 1 tbsp. smoked paprika

Directions:

1. Combine all the **Ingredients** in your Instant Pot, set on Stew for 15 minutes.
2. Release the pressure naturally and serve.

Nutrition: 320 Calories; 11g Carbohydrates; 23g Fat

Chili Sin Carne

Preparation Time: 15 minutes

Cooking Time: 35 minutes

Servings: *2*

Ingredients:

- 3 cups mixed cooked beans
- 2 cups chopped tomatoes
- 1 tbsp. yeast extract
- 2 squares very dark chocolate
- 1 tbsp. red chili flakes

Directions:

1. Combine all the Ingredients in your Instant Pot, cook for 35 minutes.
2. Release the pressure naturally and serve.

Nutrition: 240 Calories; 20g Carbohydrates; 3g Fat

Chick Pea and Kale Dish

Preparation Time: 10 minutes

Cooking Time: 25-30 minutes

Servings:*4*

Ingredients:

- 2 cups chickpea flour
- 1/2 cup green bell pepper, diced
- 1/2 cup onions, minced
- 1 tablespoon oregano
- 1 tablespoon salt
- 1 teaspoon cayenne
- 4 cups spring water
- 2 tablespoons Grape Seed Oil

Directions:

1. Boil spring water in a large pot

2. Lower heat into medium and whisk in chickpea flour

3. Add some minced onions, diced green bell pepper, seasoning to the pot and cook for 10 minutes

4. Cover dish using a baking sheet, grease with oil

5. Pour batter into the sheet and spread with a spatula

6. Cover with another sheet

7. Transfer to a fridge and chill, for 20 minutes

8. Remove from freezer and cut batter into fry shapes

9. Preheat the Air Fryer, to 385 degrees F

10. Transfer fries into the cooking basket, lightly greased and cover with parchment

11. Bake for about 15 minutes, flip and bake for 10 minutes more until golden brown

12. Serve and enjoy!

Nutrition: Calories: 271 kcal; Carbohydrates: 28 g; Fat: 15 g; Protein: 9 g

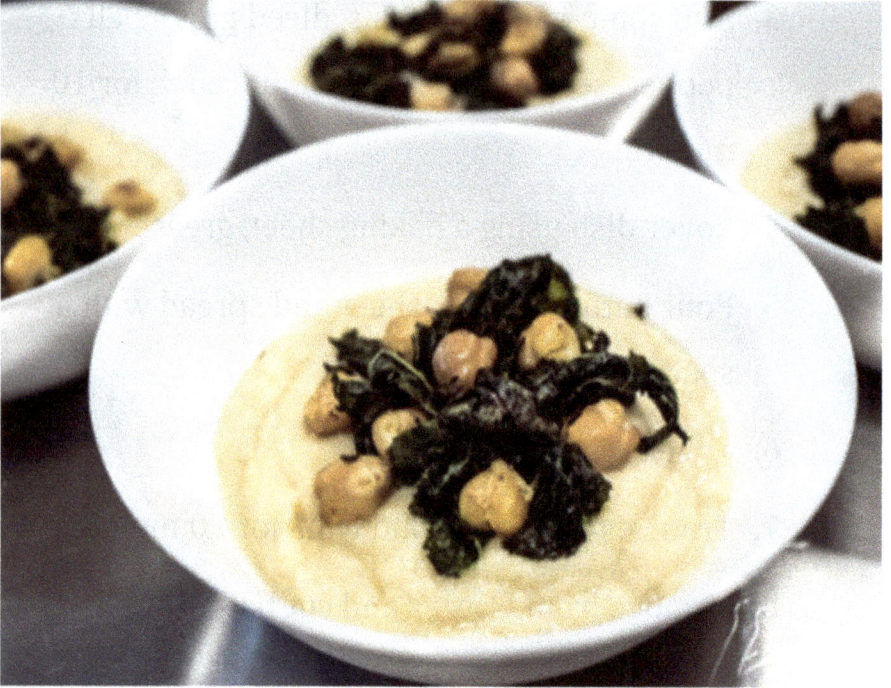

Zucchini Chips

Preparation Time: *10 minutes*

Cooking Time*: 12-15 minutes*

Servings:4

Ingredients:

- *Salt as needed*

- *Grape seed oil as needed*

- *6 zucchinis*

Directions:

1. Into 330 F, pre heat the Air Fryer

2. Wash zucchini, slice zucchini into thin strips

3. Put slices in a bowl and add oil, salt, and toss

4. Spread over the cooking basket, fry for 12-15 minutes

5. Serve and enjoy!

Nutrition: Calories: 92 kcal; Carbohydrates: 6 g;Fat: 7 g; Protein: 2 g

Classic Blueberry Spelt Muffins

Preparation Time: 10 minutes

Cooking Time: 12-15 minutes

Servings:*4*

Ingredients:

- 1/4 sea salt
- 1/3 cup maple syrup
- 1 teaspoon baking powder
- 1/2 cup sea moss
- 3/4 cup spelt flour
- 3/4 cup Kamut flour
- 1 cup hemp milk
- 1 cup blueberries

Directions:

1. Into 380 degrees F pre heat Air Fryer
2. Take your muffin tins and gently grease them

3. Take a bowl and add flour, syrup, salt, baking powder, seamless and mix well

4. Add milk and mix well

5. Fold in blueberries

6. Pour into muffin tins

7. Transfer to the cooking basket, bake for 20-25 minutes until nicely baked

8. Serve and enjoy!

Nutrition: Calories: 217 kcal; Carbohydrates: 32 g; Fat: 9 g; Protein: 4 g

Genuine Healthy Crackers

Preparation Time: 10 minutes

Cooking Time: 12-15 minutes

Servings:*4*

Ingredients:

- 1/2 cup Rye flour

- 1 cup spelt flour

- 2 teaspoons sesame seed

- 1 teaspoon agave syrup

- 1 teaspoon salt

- 2 tablespoons grapeseed oil

- 3/4 cup spring water

Directions:

1. Into 330 degrees F, Preheat the Air Fryer

2. Take a medium bowl and add all Ingredients, mix well

3. Make dough ball

4. Prepare a place for rolling out the dough, cover with a piece of parchment

5. Lightly grease paper with grape seed oil, place dough

6. Roll out, dough with a rolling pin, add more flour if needed

7. Take a shape cutter and cut dough into squares

8. Place squares in Air Fryer cooking basket

9. Brush with more oil

10.   Sprinkle salt

11.   Bake for 10-15 minutes until golden

12.   Let it cool, serve, and enjoy!

Nutrition: Calories: 226 kcal; Carbohydrates: 41 g; Fat: 3 g; Protein: 11 g

Tortilla Chips

Preparation Time: 10 minutes

Cooking Time: 8-12 minutes

Servings: *4*

Ingredients:

- 2 cups of spelt flour
- 1 teaspoon of salt
- 1/2 cup of spring water
- 1/3 cup of grapeseed oil

Directions:

1. Preheat your Air Fryer into 320 degrees F
2. Take the food processor then add salt, flour, and process well for 15 seconds
3. Gradually add grapeseed oil until mixed
4. Keep mixing until you have a nice dough

5. Formulate work surface and cover in a piece of parchment, sprinkle flour

6. Knead the dough for 1-2 minutes

7. Grease cooking basket with oil

8. Transfer dough on the cooking basket, brush oil and sprinkle salt

9. Cut dough into 8 triangles

10.   Bake for about 8-12 minutes until golden brown

11.   Serve and enjoy once done!

Nutrition: Calories: 288 kcal; Carbohydrates: 18 g; Fat: 17 g; Protein: 16 g

Pumpkin Spice Crackers

Preparation Time: 10 minutes

Cooking Time: 60 minutes

Servings: 6

Ingredients:

- 1/3 cup coconut flour
- 2 tablespoons pumpkin pie spice
- ¾ cup sunflower seeds
- ¾ cup flaxseed
- 1/3 cup sesame seeds
- 1 tablespoon ground psyllium husk powder
- 1 teaspoon sea salt
- 3 tablespoons coconut oil, melted
- 11/3 cups alkaline water

Directions:

1. Set your oven to 300 degrees F.

2. Combine all dry Ingredients in a bowl.

3. Add water and oil to the mixture and mix well.

4. Let the dough stay for 2 to 3 minutes.

5. Spread the dough evenly on a cookie sheet lined with parchment paper.

6. Bake for 30 minutes.

7. Reduce the oven heat to low and bake for another 30 minutes.

8. Crack the bread into bite-size pieces.

9. Serve

Nutrition: Calories 248; Total Fat 15.7 g; Saturated Fat 2.7 g; Cholesterol 75 mg; Sodium 94 mg; Total Carbs 0.4 g; Fiber 0g; Sugar 0 g; Protein 24.9 g

Spicy Roasted Nuts

Preparation Time: 10 minutes

Cooking Time: 15 minutes

Servings: *4*

Ingredients:

- 8 oz. pecans or almonds or walnuts
- 1 teaspoon sea salt
- 1 tablespoon olive oil or coconut oil
- 1 teaspoon ground cumin
- 1 teaspoon paprika powder or chili powder

Directions:

1. Add all the Ingredients to a skillet.
2. Roast the nuts until golden brown.
3. Serve and enjoy.

Nutrition: Calories 287; Total Fat 29.5 g; Saturated Fat 3 g; Cholesterol 0 mg; Total Carbs 5.9 g; Sugar 1.4g; Fiber 4.3 g; Sodium 388 mg; Protein 4.2 g

Wheat Crackers

Preparation Time: 10 minutes

Cooking Time: 20 minutes

Servings: *4*

Ingredients:

- 1 3/4 cups almond flour
- 1 1/2 cups coconut flour
- 3/4 teaspoon sea salt
- 1/3 cup vegetable oil
- 1 cup alkaline water
- Sea salt for sprinkling

Directions:

1. Set your oven to 350 degrees F.
2. Mix coconut flour, almond flour and salt in a bowl.

3. Stir in vegetable oil and water. Mix well until smooth.

4. Spread this dough on a floured surface into a thin sheet.

5. Cut small squares out of this sheet.

6. Arrange the dough squares on a baking sheet lined with parchment paper.

7. For about 20 minutes, bake until light golden in color.

8. Serve.

Nutrition: Calories 64; Total Fat 9.2 g; Saturated Fat 2.4 g; Cholesterol 110 mg; Sodium 276 mg; Total Carbs 9.2 g; Fiber 0.9 g; Sugar 1.4 g; Protein 1.5 g

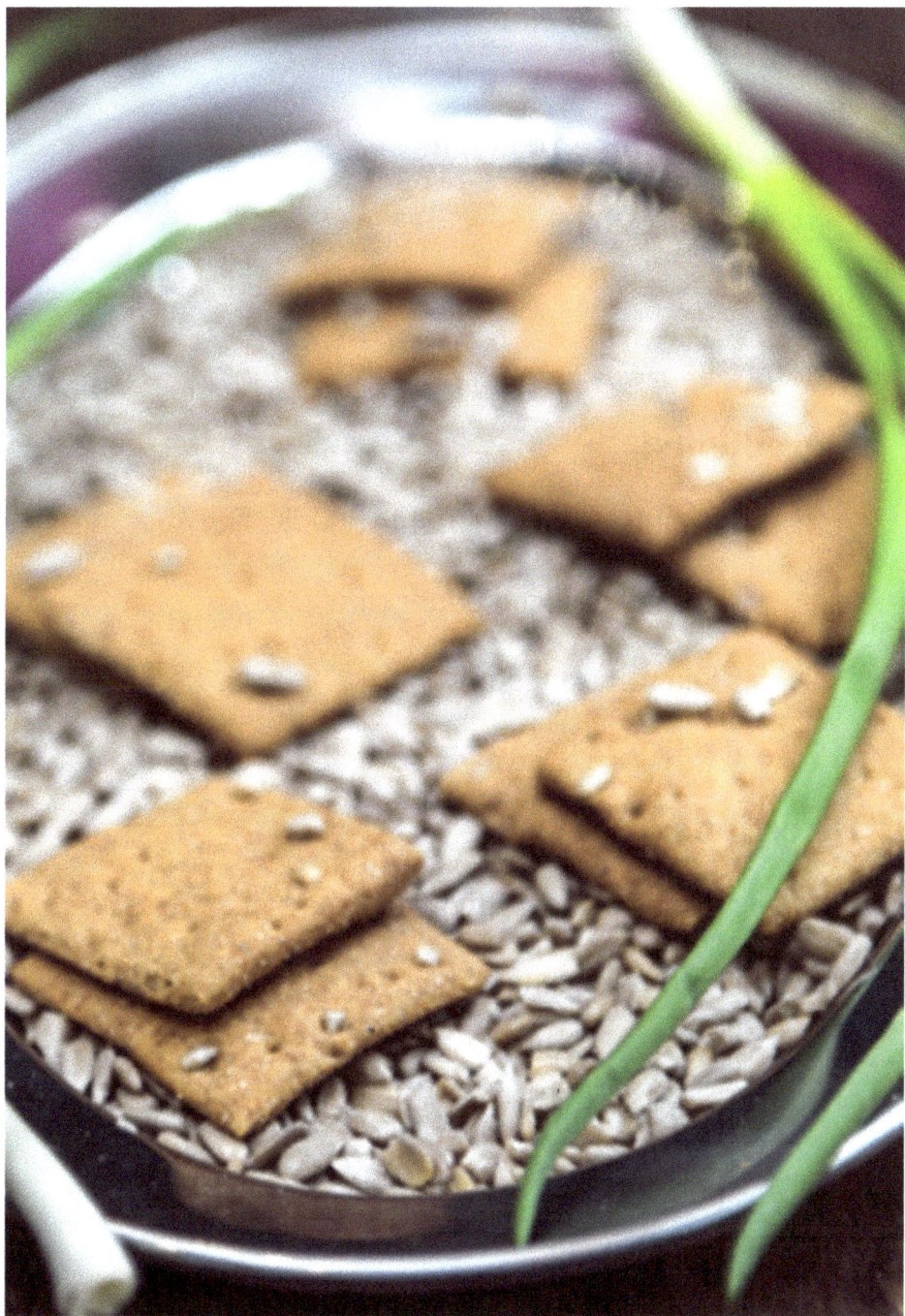

Potato Chips

Preparation Time: 10 minutes

Cooking Time: 20 minutes

Servings: *4*

Ingredients:

- 1 tablespoon vegetable oil
- 1 potato, sliced paper thin
- Sea salt, to taste

Directions:

1. Toss potato with oil and sea salt.
2. Spread the slices in a baking dish in a single layer.
3. Cook in a microwave for 5 minutes until golden brown.
4. Serve.

Nutrition: Calories 80; Total Fat 3.5 g; Saturated Fat 0.1 g; Cholesterol 320 mg; Sodium 350 mg; Total Carbs 11.6 g; Fiber 0.7 g; Sugar 0.7 g; Protein 1.2 g

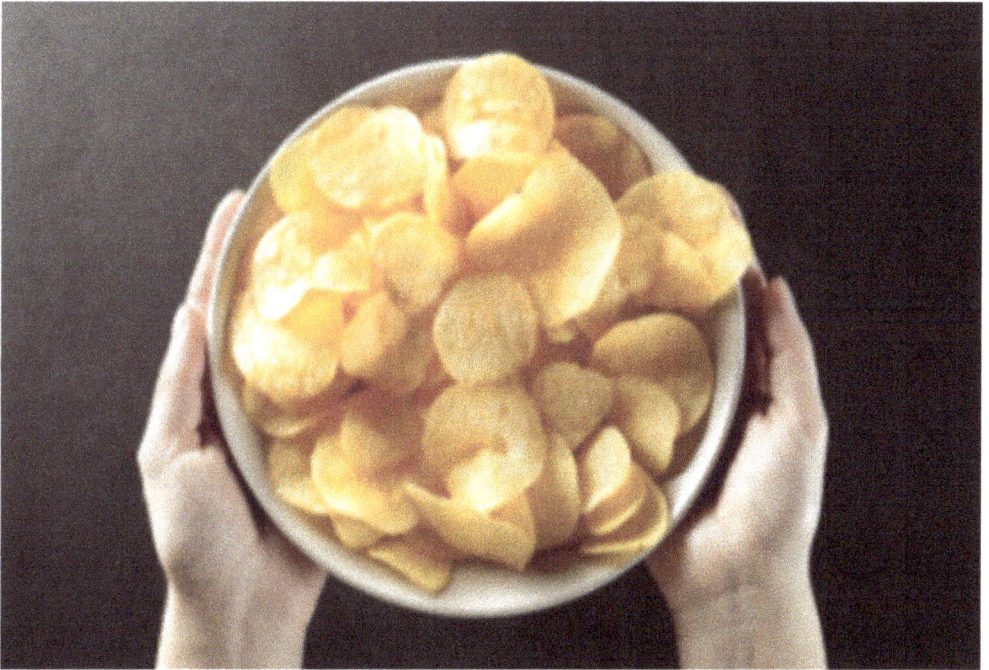

Zucchini Pepper Chips

Preparation Time: 10 minutes

Cooking Time: 15 minutes

Servings: 4

Ingredients:

- 1 2/3 cups vegetable oil

- 1 teaspoon garlic powder

- 1 teaspoon onion powder

- 1/2 teaspoon black pepper

- 3 tablespoons crushed red pepper flakes

- 2 zucchinis, thinly sliced

Directions:

1. Mix oil with all the spices in a bowl.

2. Add zucchini slices and mix well.

3. Transfer the mixture to a Ziplock bag and seal it.

4. Refrigerate for 10 minutes.

5. Spread the zucchini slices on a greased baking sheet.

6. Bake for 15 minutes

7. Serve.

Nutrition: Calories 172; Total Fat 11.1 g; Saturated Fat 5.8 g; Cholesterol 610 mg; Sodium 749 mg; Total Carbs 19.9 g; Fiber 0.2 g; Sugar 0.2 g; Protein 13.5 g

Apple Chips

Preparation Time: 5 minutes

Cooking Time: 45 minutes

Servings: 4

Ingredients:

- 2 Golden Delicious apples, cored and thinly sliced
- 1 1/2 teaspoons white sugar
- 1/2 teaspoon ground cinnamon

Directions:

1. Set your oven to 225 degrees F.
2. Place apple slices on a baking sheet.
3. Sprinkle sugar an
4. d cinnamon over apple slices.
5. Bake for 45 minutes.
6. Serve

Nutrition: Calories 127; Total Fat 3.5 g; Saturated Fat 0.5 g; Cholesterol 162 mg; Sodium 142 mg; Total Carbs 33.6g; Fiber 0.4 g; Sugar 0.5 g; Protein 4.5 g

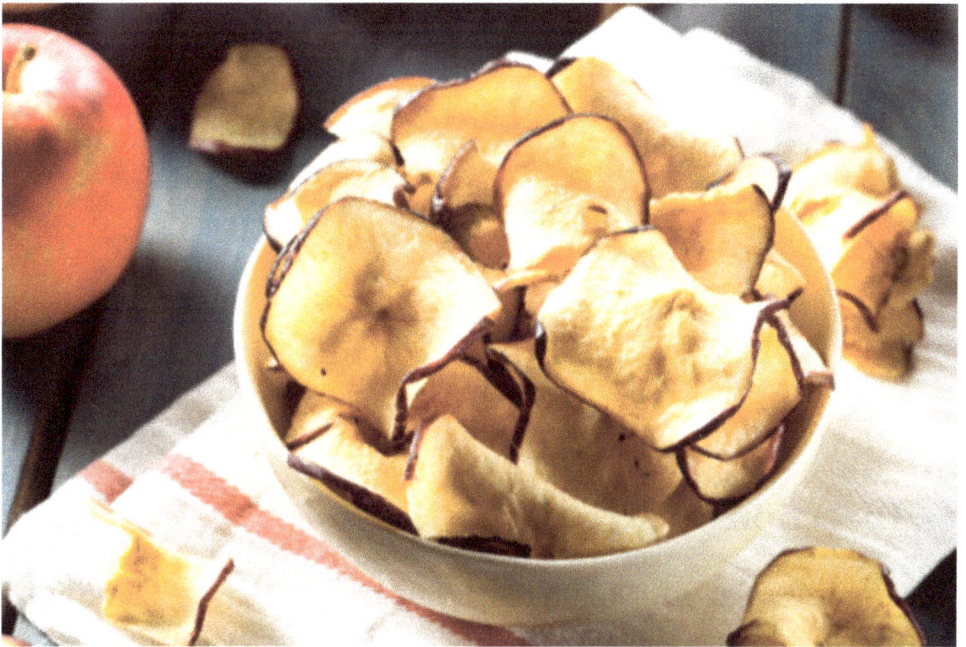

Kale Crisps

Preparation Time: 10 minutes

Cooking Time: 10 minutes

Servings: *4*

Ingredients:

- 1 bunch kale, remove the stems, leaves torn into even pieces
- 1 tablespoon olive oil
- 1 teaspoon sea salt

Directions:

1. Set your oven to 350 degrees F. Layer a baking sheet with parchment paper.
2. Spread the kale leaves on a paper towel to absorb all the moisture.
3. Toss the leaves with sea salt, and olive oil.

4. Kindly spread them, on the baking sheet and bake for 10 minutes.

5. Serve.

Nutrition: Calories 113; Total Fat 7.5 g; Saturated Fat 1.1 g; Cholesterol 20 mg; Sodium 97 mg; Total Carbs 1.4 g; Fiber 0 g; Sugar 0 g; Protein 1.1g

Carrot Chips

Preparation Time: 5 minutes

Cooking Time: 12 minutes

Servings: 4

Ingredients:

- 4 carrots, washed, peeled and sliced

- 2 teaspoons extra-virgin olive oil

- 1/4 teaspoon sea salt

Directions:

1. Set your oven to 350 degrees F.

2. Toss carrots with salt and olive oil.

3. Spread the slices into two baking sheets in a single layer.

4. Bake for 6 minutes on upper and lower rack of the oven.

5. Switch the baking racks and bake for another 6 minutes.

6. Serve.

Nutrition: Calories 153; Total Fat 7.5 g; Saturated Fat 1.1 g; Cholesterol 20 mg; Sodium 97 mg; Total Carbs 20.4 g; Fiber 0 g; Sugar 0 g; Protein 3.1g

Pita Chips

Preparation Time: 5 minutes

Cooking Time: 12 minutes

Servings: 4

Ingredients:

- 12 pita bread pockets, sliced into triangles
- 1/2 cup olive oil
- 1/2 teaspoon ground black pepper
- 1 teaspoon garlic salt
- 1/2 teaspoon dried basil
- 1 teaspoon dried chervil

Directions:

1. Set your oven to 400 degrees F.
2. Toss pita with all the remaining Ingredients in a bowl.

3. Spread the seasoned triangles on a baking sheet.

4. Bake for 7 minutes until golden brown.

5. Serve with your favorite hummus.

Nutrition: Calories 201; Total Fat 5.5 g; Saturated Fat 2.1 g; Cholesterol 10 mg; Sodium 597 mg; Total Carbs 2.4 g; Fiber 0 g; Sugar 0 g; Protein 3.1g

Sweet Potato Chips

Preparation Time: 5 minutes

Cooking Time*: 5 minutes*

Servings: *4*

Ingredients:

- 1 sweet potato, thinly sliced

- 2 teaspoons olive oil, or as needed

- Coarse sea salt, to taste

Directions:

1. Toss sweet potato with oil and salt.

2. Spread the slices in a baking dish in a single layer.

3. Cook in a microwave for 5 minutes until golden brown.

4. Serve.

Nutrition: Calories 213; Total Fat 8.5 g; Saturated Fat 3.1 g; Cholesterol 120 mg; Sodium 497 mg; Total Carbs 21.4 g; Fiber 0 g; Sugar 0 g; Protein 0.1g

Spinach and Sesame Crackers

__Preparation Time:__ 5 minutes

__Cooking Time__: 15 minutes

__Servings:__ 4

__Ingredients:__

- 2 tablespoons white sesame seeds

- 1 cup fresh spinach, washed

- 1 2/3 cups all-purpose flour

- 1/2 cup water

- 1/2 teaspoon baking powder

- 1 teaspoon olive oil

- 1 teaspoon salt

__Directions:__

1. Transfer the spinach to a blender with a half cup water and blend until smooth.

2. Add 2 tablespoons white sesame seeds, ½ teaspoon baking powder, 1 2/3 cups all-purpose flour, and 1 teaspoon salt to a bowl and stir well until combined. Add in 1 teaspoon olive oil and spinach water. Mix again and knead by using your hands until you obtain a smooth dough.

3. If the made dough is too gluey, then add more flour.

4. Using your parchment paper lightly roll out the dough as thin as possible. Cut into squares with a pizza cutter.

5. Bake into a preheated oven at 400°, for about 15to 20 minutes. Once done, let cool and then serve.

Nutrition: 223 Calories; 3g Fat; 41g Total Carbohydrates; 6g Protein

Mini Nacho Pizzas

Preparation Time: 5 minutes

Cooking Time: 10 minutes

Servings: 4

Ingredients:

- 1/4 cup refried beans, vegan

- 2 tablespoons tomato, diced

- 2 English muffins, split in half

- 1/4 cup onion, sliced

- 1/3 cup vegan cheese, shredded

- 1 small jalapeno, sliced

- 1/3 cup roasted tomato salsa

- 1/2 avocado, diced and tossed in lemon juice

Directions:

1. Add the refried beans/salsa onto the muffin bread. Sprinkle with shredded vegan cheese followed by the veggie toppings.

2. Transfer to a baking sheet and place in a preheated oven at 350 to 400 F on a top rack.

3. Put into the oven for 10 minutes and then broil for 2minutes, so that the top becomes bubbly.

4. Take out from the oven and let them cool at room temperature.

5. Top with avocado. Enjoy!

Nutrition: 133 Calories; 4.2g Fat; 719g Total Carbohydrates; 6g Protein

Pizza Sticks

Preparation Time: 10 minutes

Cooking Time: 30 minutes

Servings: 16 sticks

Ingredients:

- 5 tablespoons tomato sauce

- Few pinches of dried basil

- 1 block extra firm tofu

- 2 tablespoon + 2 teaspoon Nutritional yeast

Directions:

1. Cape the tofu in a paper tissue and put a cutting board on top, place something heavy on top and drain for about 10 to 15 minutes.

2. In the meantime, line your baking sheet with parchment paper. Cut the tofu into 16 equal pieces and place them on a baking sheet.

3. Spread each pizza stick with a teaspoon of marinara sauce.

4. Sprinkle each stick with half teaspoon of yeast, followed by basil on top.

5. Bake into a preheated oven at 425 F for about 28 to 30 minutes. Serve and enjoy!

_Nutrition:_33 Calories; 1.7g Fat; 2g Total Carbs; 3g Protein

Raw Broccoli Poppers

Preparation Time: 2 minutes

Cooking Time: 8 minutes

Servings: 4

Ingredients:

- 1/8 cup water

- 1/8 teaspoon fine sea salt

- 4 cups broccoli florets, washed and cut into 1-inch pieces

- 1/4 teaspoon turmeric powder

- 1 cup unsalted cashews, soaked overnight or at least 3-4 hours and drained

- 1/4 teaspoon onion powder

- 1 red bell pepper, seeded and

- 2 heaping tablespoons **Nutrition**al

- 2 tablespoons lemon juice

Directions:

1. Transfer the drained cashews to a high-speed blender and pulse for about 30 seconds. Add in the chopped pepper and pulse again for 30seconds.

2. Add some 2 tablespoons lemon juice, 1/8 cup water, 2heaping tablespoons **Nutrition**al yeast, ¼ teaspoon onion powder, 1/8 teaspoon fine sea salt, and 1/4 teaspoon turmeric powder. Pulse for about 45 seconds until smooth.

3. Handover the broccoli into a bowl and add in chopped cheesy cashew mixture. Toss well until coated.

4. Transfer the pieces of broccoli to the trays of a yeast dehydrator.

5. Follow the dehydrator's instructions and dehydrate for about 8 minutes at 125 F or until crunchy.

Nutrition: 408 Calories; 32g Fat; 22g Total Carbohydrates; 15g Protein

Blueberry Cauliflower

Preparation Time: 2 minutes

Cooking Time: 5 minutes

Servings: 1

Ingredients:

- ¼ cup frozen strawberries

- 2 teaspoons maple syrup

- ¾ cup unsweetened cashew milk

- 1 teaspoon vanilla extract

- ½ cup plain cashew yogurt

- 5 tablespoons powdered peanut butter

- ¾ cup frozen wild blueberries

- ½ cup cauliflower florets, coarsely chopped

Directions:

1. Add all the smoothie Ingredients to a high-speed blender.

2. Blitz to combine until smooth.

3. Pour into a chilled glass and serve.

Nutrition: 340 Calories; 11g Fat; 48g Total Carbohydrates; 16g Protein

Candied Ginger

Preparation Time: 10 minutes

Cooking Time: 40 minutes

Servings: 3 to 5

Ingredients:

- 2 1/2 cups salted pistachios, shelled

- 1 1/4 teaspoons powdered ginger

- 3 tablespoons pure maple syrup

Directions:

1. Add 1 1/4 teaspoons powdered ginger to a bowl with pistachios. Stir well until combined. There

2. should be no lumps.

3. Drizzle with 3 tablespoons of maple syrup and stir well.

4. Transfer to a baking sheet lined with parchment paper and spread evenly.

5. Cook into a preheated oven at 275 F for about 20 minutes.

6. Take out from oven, stir, and cook for further 10 to 15 minutes.

7. Let it cool for about few minutes until crispy. Enjoy!

Nutrition: 378 Calories; 27.6g Fat; 26g Total Carbohydrates; 13g Protein

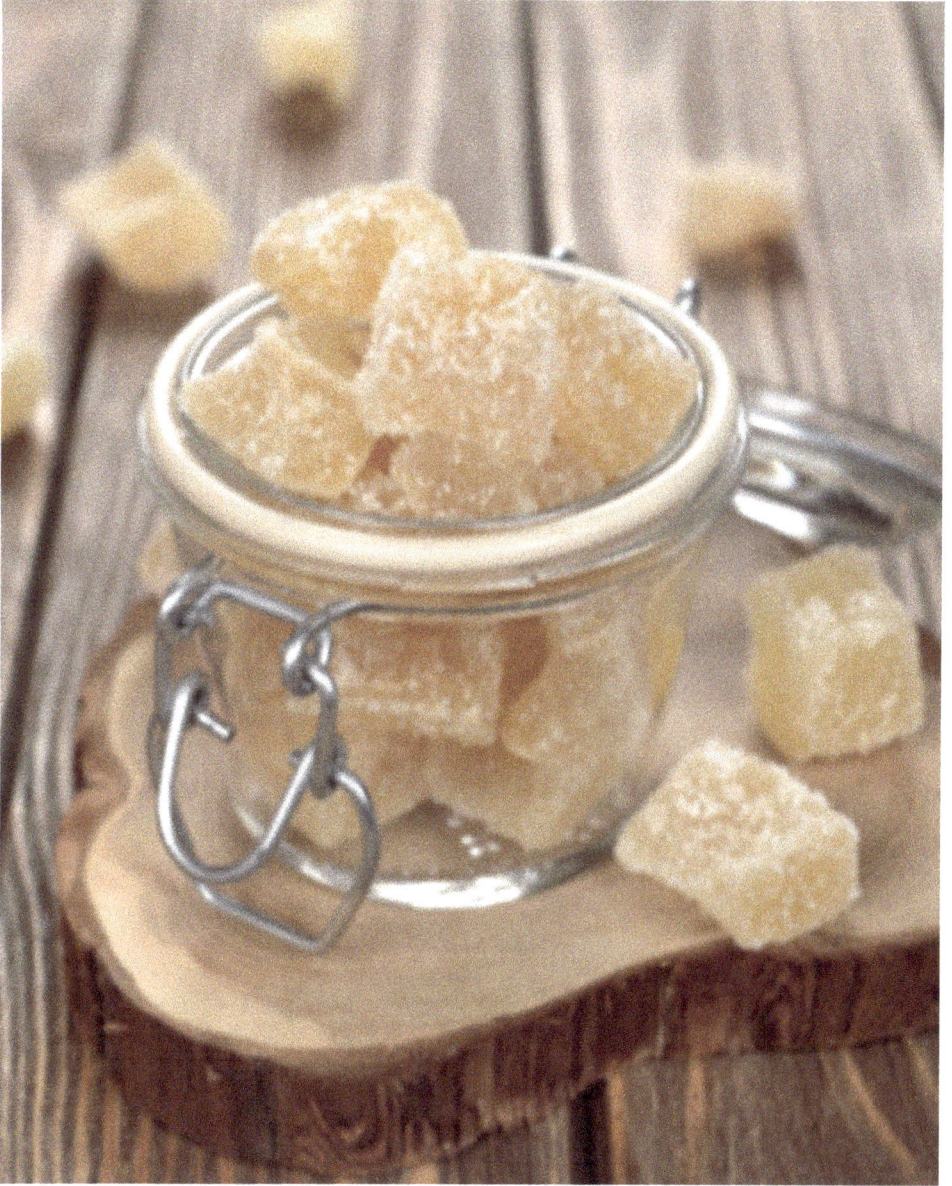

Chia Crackers

Preparation Time: 20 minutes

Cooking Time: 1 hour

Servings: 24-26 crackers

Ingredients:

- 1/2 cup pecans, chopped

- 1/2 cup chia seeds

- 1/2 teaspoon cayenne pepper

- 1 cup water

- 1/4 cup **Nutrition**al yeast

- 1/2 cup pumpkin seeds

- 1/4 cup ground flax

- Salt and pepper, to taste

Directions:

1. Mix around 1/2 cup chia seeds and 1 cup water. Keep it aside.

2. Take another bowl and combine all the remaining **Ingredients** . Combine well and stir in the chia water mixture until you obtained dough.

3. Transfer the dough onto a baking sheet and rollout (¼" thick).

4. Transfer into a preheated oven at 325ºF and bake for about half an hour.

5. Take out from the oven, flip over the dough, and cut it into desired cracker shape/squares.

6. Spread and back again for further half an hour, or until crispy and browned.

7. Once done, take out from oven and let them cool at room temperature. Enjoy!

Nutrition: 41 calories; 3.1g Fat; 2g Total Carbohydrates; 2g Protein

Orange- Spiced Pumpkin Hummus

Preparation Time: 2 minutes

Cooking Time: 5 minutes

Servings: 4 cups

Ingredients:

- 1 tablespoon maple syrup

- 1/2 teaspoon salt

- 1 can (16oz.) garbanzo beans,

- 1/8 teaspoon ginger or nutmeg

- 1 cup canned pumpkin Blend,

- 1/8 teaspoon cinnamon

- 1/4 cup tahini

- 1 tablespoon fresh orange juice

- Pinch of orange zest, for garnish

- 1 tablespoon apple cider vinegar

Directions:

1. Mix all the **Ingredients** to a food processor blender and blend until slightly chunky.

2. Serve right away and enjoy!

Nutrition: 291 Calories; 22.9g Fat; 15g Total Carbohydrates; 12g Protein

Cinnamon Maple Sweet Potato Bites

__Preparation Time:__ 5 minutes

__Cooking Time__: 25 minutes

__Servings:__ 3 to 4

__Ingredients:__

- ½ teaspoon corn-starch

- 1 teaspoon cinnamon

- 4 medium sweet potatoes, then peeled, and cut into bite-size cubes

- 2 to 3 tablespoons maple syrup

- 3 tablespoons butter, melted

__Directions:__

1. Transfer the potato cubes to a Ziploc bag and add in 3 tablespoons of melted butter. Seal and

shake well until the potato cubes are coated with butter.

2. Add in the remaining Ingredients and shake again.

3. Transfer the potato cubes to a parchment-lined baking sheet. Cubes shouldn't be stacked on one another.

4. Sprinkle with cinnamon, if needed, and bake in a preheated oven at 425°F for about 25 to 30 minutes, stirring once during cooking.

5. Once done, take them out and stand at room temperature. Enjoy!

6.

Nutrition: 436 Calories; 17.4g Fat; 71.8g Total Carbohydrates; 4.1g Protein

Cheesy Kale Chips

Preparation Time: 3 minutes

Cooking Time: 12 minutes

Servings: 4

Ingredients:

- 3 tablespoons **Nutrition**al yeast
- 1 head curly kale, washed, ribs
- 3/4 teaspoon garlic powder
- 1 tablespoon olive oil
- 1 teaspoon onion powder
- Salt, to taste

Directions:

1. Line cookie sheets with parchment paper.
2. Drain the kale leaves and spread on a paper removed and leaves torn into chip-

3. towel. Then, kindly transfer the leaves to a bowl and sized pieces

4. add in 1 teaspoon onion powder, 3 tablespoons **Nutrition**al yeast, 1 tablespoon olive oil, and 3/4

5. teaspoon garlic powder. Mix with your hands.

6. Spread the kale onto prepared cookie sheets. They shouldn't touch each other.

7. Bake into a preheated oven for about 350 F for about 10to 12 minutes.

8. Once crisp, take out from the oven, and sprinkle with a bit of salt. Serve and enjoy!

__Nutrition:__ 71 Calories; 4g Fat; 5g Total Carbohydrates; 4g Protein

Lemon Roasted Bell Pepper

Preparation Time: 10 minutes

Cooking Time: 5 minutes

Servings: *4*

Ingredients:

- 4 bell peppers

- 1 teaspoon olive oil

- 1 tablespoon mango juice

- 1/4 teaspoon garlic, minced

- 1 teaspoons oregano

- 1 pinch salt

- 1 pinch pepper

Directions:

1. Start heating the Air Fryer to 390 degrees F

2. Place some bell pepper in the Air fryer

3. Drizzle it with the olive oil and air fry for 5 minutes

4. Take a **Serving** plate and transfer it

5. Take a small bowl and add garlic, oregano, mango juice, salt, and pepper

6. Mix them well and drizzle the mixture over the peppers

7. Serve and enjoy!

__Nutrition:__ Calories: 59 kcal; Carbohydrates: 6 g; Fat: 5 g; Protein: 4 g

Subtle Roasted Mushrooms

Preparation Time: 10 minutes

Cooking Time: 5 minutes

Servings:4

Ingredients:

- 2 teaspoons mixed Sebi Friendly herbs
- 1 tablespoon olive oil
- 1/2 teaspoon garlic powder
- 2 pounds mushrooms
- 2 tablespoons date sugar

Directions:

1. Wash mushrooms and turn dry in a plate of mixed greens spinner
2. Quarter them and put in a safe spot
3. Put garlic, oil, and spices in the dish of your oar type air fryer

4. Warmth for 2 minutes

5. Stir it.

6. Add some mushrooms and cook 25 minutes

7. Then include vermouth and cook for 5 minutes more

8. Serve and enjoy!

Nutrition: Calories: 94 kcal; Carbohydrates: 3 g; Fat: 8 g; Protein: 2 g

Fancy Spelt Bread

Preparation Time: 10 minutes

Cooking Time: 5 minutes

Servings:*4*

Ingredients:

- 1 cup spring water
- 1/2 cup of coconut milk
- 3 tablespoons avocado oil
- 1 teaspoon baking soda
- 1 tablespoon agave nectar
- 4 and 1/2 cups spelt flour
- 1 and 1/2 teaspoon salt

Directions:

1. Pre-heat your Air Fryer to 355 degrees F
2. Take a big bowl and add baking soda, salt, flour whisk well

3. Add 3/4 cup of water, plus coconut milk, oil and mix well

4. Sprinkle your working surface with flour, add dough to the flour

5. Roll well

6. Knead for about three minutes, adding small amounts of flour until dough is a nice ball

7. Place parchment paper in your cooking basket

8. Lightly grease your pan and put the dough inside

9. Transfer into Air Fryer and bake for 30-45 minutes until done

10. Remove then insert a stick to check for doneness

11. If done already serve and enjoy, if not, let it cook for a few minutes more

Nutrition: Calories: 203 kcal; Carbohydrates: 37 g; Fat: 4g; Protein: 7 g

Crispy Crunchy Hummus

Preparation Time: 10 minutes

Cooking Time: 10-15 minutes

Servings:*4*

Ingredients:

- 1/2 a red onion
- 2 tablespoons fresh coriander
- 1/4 cup cherry tomatoes
- 1/2 a red bell pepper
- 1 tablespoon dulse flakes
- Juice of lime
- Salt to taste
- 3 tablespoons olive oil
- 2 tablespoons tahini
- 1 cup warm chickpeas

Directions:

1. Prepare your Air Fryer cooking basket

2. Add chickpeas to your cooking container and cook for 10-15 minutes, making a point to continue blending them every once in a while, until they are altogether warmed

3. Add warmed chickpeas to a bowl and include tahini, salt, lime

4. Utilize a fork to pound chickpeas and fixings in a glue until smooth

5. Include hacked onion, cherry tomatoes, ringer pepper, dulse drops, and olive oil

6. Blend well until consolidated

7. Serve hummus with a couple of cuts of spelt bread

Nutrition: Calories: 95 kcal; Carbohydrates: 5 g; Fat: 5 g; Protein: 5 g

Dill Celery Soup

__Preparation Time:__ 10 minutes

__Cooking Time__: 30 minutes

Servings: 4

Ingredients:

- 6 cups celery stalk, chopped
- 2 cups filtered alkaline water
- 1 medium onion, chopped
- 1/2 tsp. dill
- 1 cup of coconut milk
- 1/4 tsp. sea salt

Directions:

1. Combine all elements into the direct pot and mix fine.
2. Cover pot with lid and select soup mode it takes 30 minutes.

3. Release pressure using the quick release **Directions:** than open lid carefully.

4. Blend the soup utilizing a submersion blender until smooth.

5. Stir well and serve.

__Nutrition:__ Calories 193; Fat 15.3 g; Carbohydrates 10.9 g; Protein 5.2 g; Sugar 5.6 g; Cholesterol 0 mg

Creamy Avocado-Broccoli Soup

Preparation Time: 10 minutes

Cooking Time: 15 minutes

Servings: 1-2

Ingredients:

- 2-3 flowers broccoli

- 1 small avocado

- 1 yellow onion

- 1 green or red pepper

- 1 celery stalk

- 2 cups vegetable broth (yeast-free)

- Celtic Sea Salt to taste

Directions:

1. Warmth vegetable stock (don't bubble).
   Include hacked onion and broccoli, and warm

for a few minutes. At that point put in blender, include the avocado, pepper and celery and Blend until the soup is smooth (include some more water whenever wanted). Flavor and serve warm. Delicious!!

Nutrition: Calories: 60g; Carbohydrates: 11g; Fat: 2 g; Protein: 2g

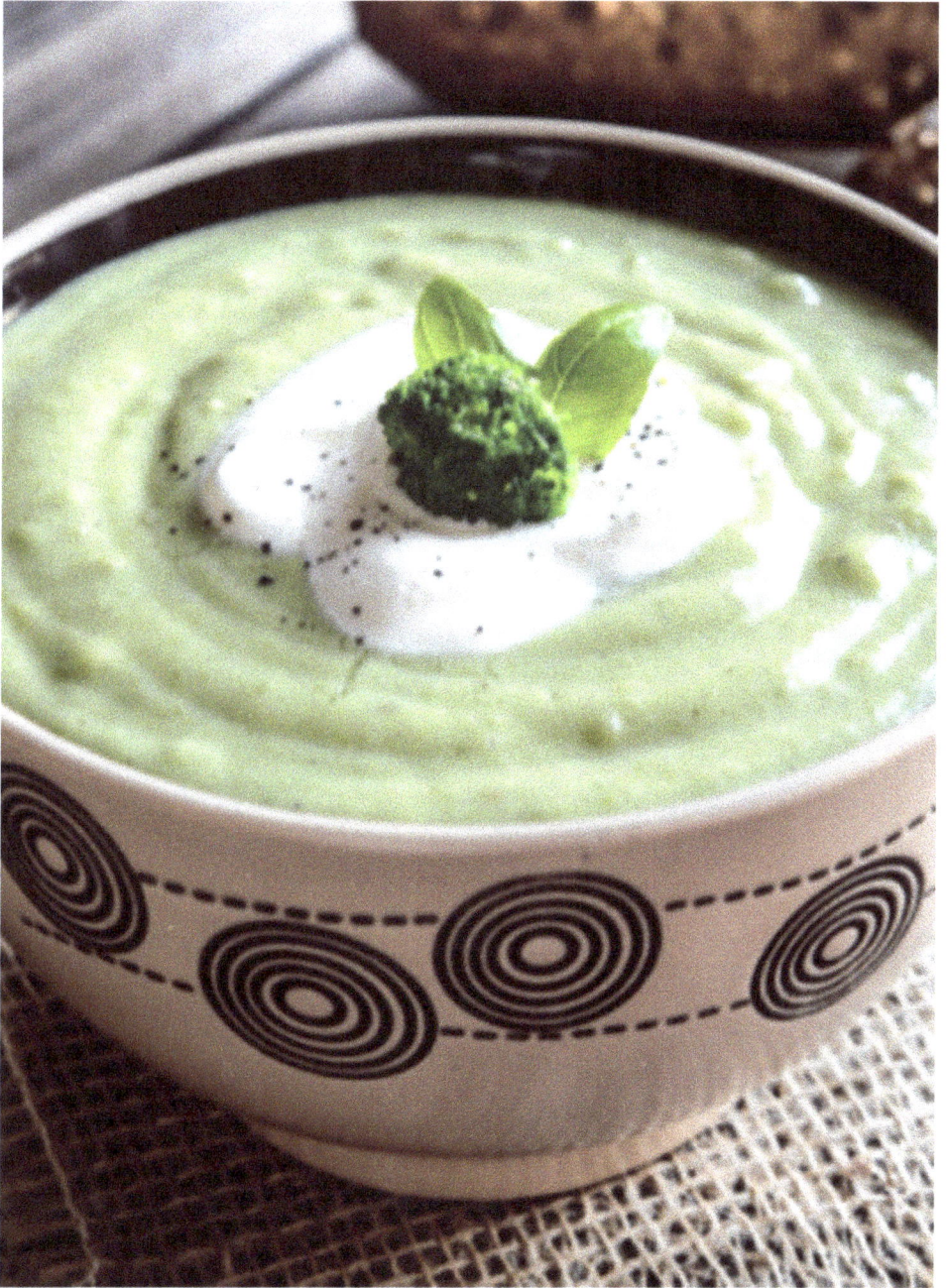

Fresh Garden Vegetable Soup

**Preparation Time:** 7 minutes

**Cooking Time**: 20 minutes

Servings: 1-2

**Ingredients:**

- 2 huge carrots

- 1 little zucchini

- 1 celery stem

- 1 cup of broccoli

- 3 stalks of asparagus

- 1 yellow onion

- 1 quart of (antacid) water

- 4-5 tsps. Of sans yeast vegetable stock

- 1 tsp. new basil

- 2 tsps. Ocean salt to taste

Directions:

1. Put water in pot, include the vegetable stock just as the onion and bring to bubble.

2. In the meantime, cleave the zucchini, the broccoli and the asparagus, and shred the carrots and the celery stem in a food processor.

3. When the water is bubbling, it would be ideal if you turn off the oven as we would prefer not to heat up the vegetables. Simply put them all in the high temp water and hold up until the vegetables arrive at wanted delicacy.

4. Permit to cool somewhat, at that point put all fixings into blender and blend until you get a thick, smooth consistency.

Nutrition: Calories: 43; Carbohydrates: 7g; Fat: 1 g

Raw Some Gazpacho Soup

Preparation Time: 7 minutes

Cooking Time: 3 hours

Servings: 3-4

Ingredients:

- 500g tomatoes

- 1 small cucumber

- 1 red pepper

- 1 onion

- 2 cloves of garlic

- 1 small chili

- 1 quart of water (preferably alkaline water)

- 4 tbsp. cold-pressed olive oil

- Juice of one fresh lemon

- 1 dash of cayenne pepper

- Sea salt to taste

Directions:

1. Remove the skin of the cucumber and cut all vegetables in large pieces.

2. Put all Ingredients except the olive oil in a blender and mix until smooth.

3. Add the olive oil and mix again until oil is emulsified.

4. Put the soup in the fridge and chill for at least 2 hours (soup should be served ice cold).

5. Add some salt and pepper to taste, mix, place the soup in bowls, garnish with chopped scallions, cucumbers, tomatoes and peppers and enjoy!

Nutrition: Calories: 39; Carbohydrates: 8g; Fat: 0.5 g; Protein: 0.2g

Alkaline Carrot Soup with Fresh Mushrooms

Preparation Time: 10 minutes

Cooking Time: 20 minutes

Servings: 1-2

Ingredients:

- 4 mid-sized carrots

- 4 mid-sized potatoes

- 10 enormous new mushrooms (champignons or chanterelles)

- 1/2 white onion

- 2 tbsp. olive oil (cold squeezed, additional virgin)

- 3 cups vegetable stock

- 2 tbsp. parsley, new and cleaved

- Salt and new white pepper

Directions:

1. Wash and strip carrots and potatoes and dice them.

2. Warm up vegetable stock in a pot on medium heat. Cook carrots and potatoes for around 15 minutes. Meanwhile finely shape onion and braise them in a container with olive oil for around 3 minutes.

3. Wash mushrooms, slice them to wanted size and add to the container, cooking approx. an additional 5 minutes, blending at times. Blend carrots, vegetable stock and potatoes, and put substance of the skillet into pot.

4. When nearly done, season with parsley, salt and pepper and serve hot. Appreciate this alkalizing soup!

Nutrition: Calories: 75; Carbohydrates: 13g; Fat: 1.8g; Protein: 1 g

Swiss Cauliflower-Omental-Soup

__Preparation Time:__ 10 minutes

__Cooking Time__: 15 minutes

__Servings:__ 3-4

Ingredients:

- 2 cups cauliflower pieces

- 1 cup potatoes, cubed

- 2 cups vegetables stock (without yeast)

- 3 tbsp. Swiss Omental cheddar, cubed

- 2 tbsp. new chives

- 1 tbsp. pumpkin seeds

- 1 touch of nutmeg and cayenne pepper

Directions:

1. Cook cauliflower and potato in vegetable stock until delicate and Blend with a blender.

2. Season the soup with nutmeg and cayenne, and possibly somewhat salt and pepper.

3. Include Emmenthal cheddar and chives and mix a couple of moments until the soup is smooth and prepared to serve. Enhance it with pumpkin seeds.

Nutrition: Calories: 65; Carbohydrates: 13g; Fat: 2g; Protein: 1g

Chilled Parsley-Gazpacho with Lime & Cucumber

Preparation Time: 10 minutes

Cooking Time: 2 hours

Servings: 1

Ingredients:

- 4-5 middle sized tomatoes

- 2 tbsp. olive oil, extra virgin and cold pressed

- 2 large cups fresh parsley

- 2 ripe avocados

- 2 cloves garlic, diced

- 2 limes, juiced

- 4 cups vegetable broth

- 1 middle sized cucumber

- 2 small red onions, diced

- 1 tsp. dried oregano

- 1½ tsp. paprika powder

- ½ tsp. cayenne pepper

- Sea salt and freshly ground pepper to taste

Directions:

1. In a pan, heat up olive oil and sauté onions and garlic until translucent. Set aside to cool down.

2. Use a large blender and blend parsley, avocado, tomatoes, cucumber, vegetable broth, lime juice and onion-garlic mix until smooth. Add some water if desired, and season with cayenne pepper, paprika powder, oregano, salt and pepper. Blend again and put in the fridge for at least 1, 5 hours.

3. Tip: Add chives or dill to the gazpacho. Enjoy this great alkaline (cold) soup!

Nutrition: Calories: 48; Carbohydrates: 12 g; Fat: 0.8g

Chilled Avocado Tomato Soup

Preparation Time: 7 minutes

Cooking Time: 20 minutes

Servings: 1-2

Ingredients:

- 2 small avocados
- 2 large tomatoes
- 1 stalk of celery
- 1 small onion
- 1 clove of garlic
- Juice of 1 fresh lemon
- 1 cup of water (best: alkaline water)
- A handful of fresh lavages
- Parsley and sea salt to taste

Directions:

1. Scoop the avocados and cut all veggies in little pieces.

2. Spot all fixings in a blender and blend until smooth.

3. Serve chilled and appreciate this nutritious and sound soluble soup formula!

Nutrition: Calories: 68; Carbohydrates: 15g; Fat: 2g; Protein: 8g

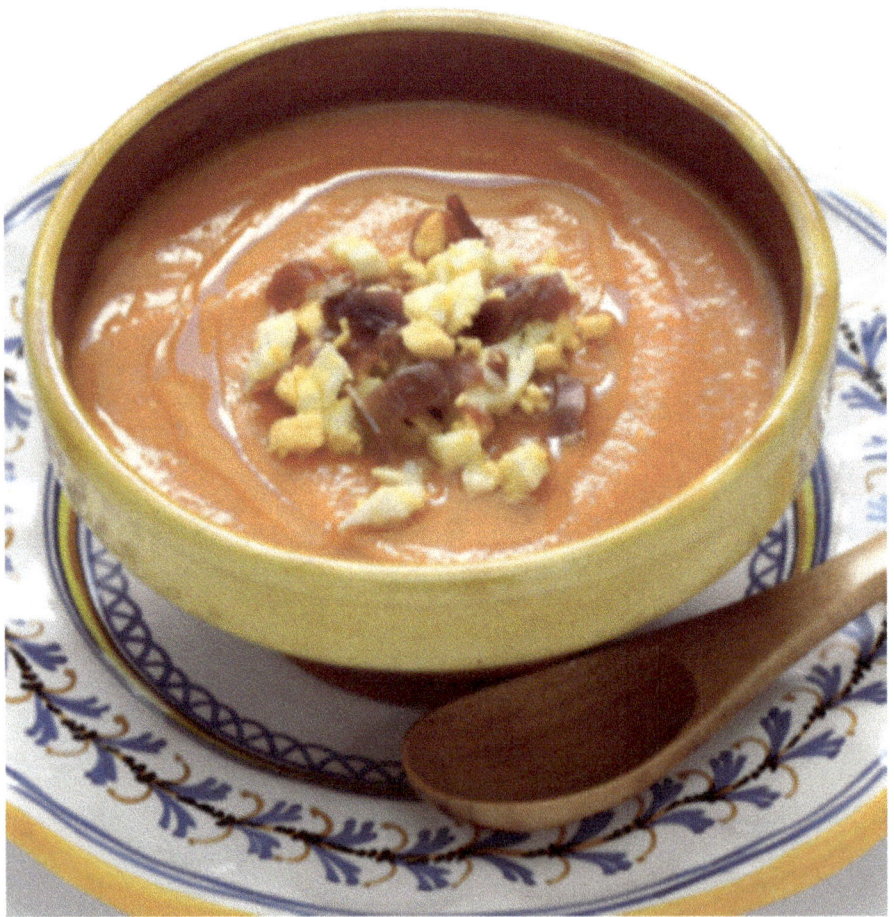

www.ingramcontent.com/pod-product-compliance
Lightning Source LLC
Chambersburg PA
CBHW050746030426
42336CB00012B/1674